A Missy Barrett Chapter Book

FANTASTIC THINGS

ELYSE BRUCE

FANTASTIC THINGS

Fantastic Things

CHAPTER 1

Missy sat on the front steps and watched her older brothers, Josh and Aaron, play one-on-one basketball in the driveway. Aaron, being the oldest brother, seemed to be trouncing Josh. By Missy's count, Aaron had racked up twice as many points as Josh.

"Josh and Aaron are the best," she rhymed in informal cheerleader rap style. "They play the game just like the rest."

Aaron stopped and turned towards Missy. "What kind of cheer is that?" he laughed. "We play the game *just like the rest*? You mean we're only as *good* as everyone else? Is that what you're saying, Missy Barrett?"

Missy shrugged her shoulders and raised her eyebrows. "Well, isn't that better than *not* being as good as the rest?" she asked innocently.

Just then, Josh zipped past Aaron, veered to one side and then to the other, finally slam dunking the ball into the net. Missy's eyes grew wide at how quickly Josh had taken advantage of Aaron's momentary lapse of attention to the game.

"Score!" Josh hollered exuberantly, followed by an awkward modified dance he'd seen football players do on television when they made it into the end field without getting tackled.

"I think that should be a do-over," Missy suggested, wanting to be fair to both players. "Aaron got distracted by my cheer."

"Nope," Josh replied cheerfully. "You snooze, you lose. Isn't that what Grandpa always says? Yes, it is, and I know how much you like repeating what Grandpa says."

Josh continued to strut up and down the driveway celebrating his tactical play in a game that had been, up to this point, severely lacking in successful strategy. Missy giggled as she watched Josh perform a dance that reminded her of how cats hurry along tin roofs on hot summer days.

"In your face, college boy," Josh taunted his big brother good-humoredly.

Aaron chuckled. "Josh, you got me. Nice play."

"But Aaron," Missy objected, "Josh got that point because I distracted you. That's not fair."

"Everything in love and war is fair," Josh hooted from the far end of the driveway where he continued to celebrate his victory. "That's something *else* Grandpa says, so yeah, the point is totally *mine!* Mark it down on the score card, Missy."

"He's right, you know," Aaron told his little sister. He brushed his hair away from his face, and Missy noticed for the first time that his cheeks were bright red.

"It doesn't matter that he scored because I got distracted. It's up to me to pay attention to sneak attacks like that. Besides," he added, "I was getting winded so maybe I'm using your cheer as an excuse to rest up a bit." He grinned broadly, and Missy relented, finally agreeing that Josh had scored the point legitimately.

Josh staggered back towards Aaron, basketball in hand once again. "As they say in the movies, nice play, old man."

"What movies have you been watching where people say that anyway?" Aaron teased his younger brother. "The 'Thin Man' movies?"

A month ago, on family movie night, Grandpa Barrett announced that he'd brought a movie with him for the family to watch. At the time, he and Josh had rolled their eyes since their grandfather, in their opinion, had dated taste. What they meant by dated taste was that it seemed to be stuck in their great-grandparents' generation of black-and-white movies of the early years of Hollywood.

This time, he'd brought a movie that he said MGM had filmed in the space of two weeks and on a B-picture budget. He'd said it was a sleeper movie because B-movies weren't expected to be popular like "The Wizard of Oz" and "Gone With The Wind." But once the movie hit theaters, this sleeper movie was an instant hit with movie goers, and pretty soon there was a string of movies and it became what studios these days call a franchise.

The movie stuck with Josh, most likely because it was wild and zany just as much as it was a murder mystery. By the time the main character was solving the mystery and exposing the criminal (which happened at a dinner party somewhere between cocktails and the first course), Josh had succumbed to the magic of the 'Thin Man' movie.

"Well, you know," Josh began, returning volley, "there's a lot to be said about how people talked back in the thirties."

"If we're going to stand around just talking, I'm going in the house to get us some lemonade," Missy announced. She suspected that both brothers were trying to find ways to catch their breath before getting back to their game. This was a perfect opportunity to get everyone (herself included) something to drink so they wouldn't get dehydrated.

"Not to worry," Aaron said, as he leapt up the front steps. "I'll go get us all something to drink. Wait here, okay?" With that he opened the door and sauntered into the house.

Josh ambled over to the front steps and dropped down beside Missy sitting on the top step.

"Wait here, he says," he joked with Missy, nudging her with his elbow. "As if we're going to disappear on him."

"Yeah, like Casper the Friendly Ghost," Missy agreed, nudging her brother back with her shoulder. "Or those two famous television magicians."

"Penn and Teller?" Josh asked, hoping he'd guessed the right two magicians. With Missy, it was always fun trying to figure out what she meant exactly.

"Yeah, those two guys," Missy confirmed, nodding her head. "The one guy is really tall, and the other guy never talks. I wonder if he ever talks. Sometimes I think maybe he doesn't talk because he's shy, and sometimes I think maybe he doesn't talk because he's like Harpo from the Marx Brothers."

"I'm pretty sure he talks, Missy," Josh assured his sister. "It's just how they decided to brand themselves and get noticed in a sea of talented magicians. I mean, after all, when they started out, they were competing for attention like all the other magicians. Know what I mean?"

"Yeah, I know what you mean."

Missy studied her brother's face carefully. Like Aaron, his face was flushed, and like Aaron, he was huffing and puffing brought on by sinking baskets and blocking plays. She wondered if he was feeling all right, mostly because Josh suffered from a very rare disease: Myasthenia Gravis.

CHAPTER 2

The day had turned out to be nicer than forecasted on the radio at breakfast. The weatherman had predicted light showers throughout the day, but it was already two in the afternoon and not a drop of rain had fallen. Missy wondered where the rain had decided to fall instead, imagining that if raindrops were animated, maybe they held a vote to decide if they should go to town or stay out where the farms were and where the rain was most needed.

"Can I ask you a question?" Missy put to her brother.

"I dunno," he answered. "Can you?"

"Josh," Missy said, annoyed that her brother had taken to using their mother's stock phrase response whenever someone asked if they could ask a question. "You know what I mean!"

"Yeah, I know what you mean," Josh replied as he ruffled Missy's hair. "Ask. If I know the answer, I'll answer. If I don't, well, I just won't."

Missy giggled. When Josh stated the obvious it never sounded like he was making fun of anyone. In fact, he sounded a bit like Dr. Henderson who knew a lot about anything medical but let patients know he didn't know everything about all things medical.

"What does fit mean?"

"Fit?" Josh repeated, puzzled by the word.

"Yeah, fit, like in the song," Missy continued.

Smiling, Josh replied, "You're going to have to give me more to go on than just that. What song?" He hoped that the song wasn't going to be one he'd never heard before otherwise Missy would have him looking it up on the Internet in minutes. *'Please make it a song I know. Please make it a song I know,'* he pleaded in his head.

"You know the one where they sing, *'Joshua fit the battle of Jericho.'* What does fit mean when it's in a sentence like that?" Missy wanted to know. "And what kind of fit makes a whole wall fall down?"

"Where'd you hear that song?" Josh asked. He'd heard the song years ago as a child, and at the time their mother had said it wasn't a song that was sung much anymore. Since it wasn't sung much anymore, he wondered where Missy had heard it.

"From the mailman," Missy said. "When he delivered the mail today, he was singing that song except not too loud so as not to bug anyone I'm guessing. I didn't want to be rude and ask him what *fit* meant, but I've been trying to figure it out and I just can't."

"Well, Missy," Josh explained talking in the long, drawn-out way he'd heard their Uncle Bob talk, "it's like this. Fit doesn't mean fit the way you think it does. It's like when people say ain't when they mean isn't, or din't when they mean didn't."

"Okay," Missy said, following along. "But that still doesn't make sense because then the song is '*Joshua fin't the battle of Jericho*' and I never heard the word *fin't* before. Have you?"

"You're getting ahead of yourself," Josh let his sister know.

"Oh, okay. Sorry about that."

"So like I was saying," Josh said, continuing where he'd left off, "fit doesn't mean fit the way you think it does. It actually means fought."

"Then why do they say fit?"

"I'm getting to that," Josh replied, realizing that Uncle Bob's way of explaining things wasn't going to work this time around. Missy wanted an immediate, to-the-point answer. "What they mean is fought as in

'*Joshua fought the battle of Jericho*.' It's just that instead of singing fought, they sing fit."

"That makes zero zip sense, Josh," Missy countered, her brow furrowed. "If fit means fought, why not sing fought instead of fit? They're both the same size – fit, fought, fit, fought."

Josh was stuck for an answer. If he didn't want to wind up stuck on the computer trying to track down the answer, he had to come up with an answer Missy would accept. He rattled his brains looking for anything that would get him out of the trap Missy had unintentionally set for him.

"I think it has to do with how people heard the song the first time the original singer sang it for them," Josh postulated, making it up as he went along. "Kind of like misheard lyrics from the olden days. That kind of thing."

This made sense to Missy, and she saw no reason to question it further. After all, if she couldn't trust her own brother to tell her the facts, who could she trust?

They sat silently for a while, watching the occasional car drive up or down the street in front of the house. A cat trotted across the front lawn and into Mrs. Whittington's yard next door, and Missy checked the livingroom window to see if Sali Dali Cat or Oreo

Speedwagon had seen the trespassing feline. They hadn't and Missy breathed easy.

Out of the blue, she said, "Remember that time when you could hardly talk and mom said it sounded like you had marbles in your mouth?"

"Which time?"

"I guess it doesn't really matter which time," Missy admitted as she looked her brother squarely in the face. "I'm just having trouble figuring out how mom knows what it sounds like to talk with marbles in your mouth."

"I dunno," Josh replied.

"Do you think maybe when she was little that somebody put marbles in their mouth and tried to talk?" Missy wondered. She couldn't imagine her mother doing something that dangerous herself, but maybe there was a wild neighborhood kid that did all kinds of crazy things just because he could.

"I think it's probably just a figure of speech, Missy," Josh said. It got him wondering though. How *did* their mother know what a mouth full of marbles sounded like?

"Probably that's it," Missy agreed. Josh's guess made sense to her. She watched the empty street for a few more seconds, and then asked, "What's it like when you talk and nobody understands you because your M.G. is making it so you can't talk right?"

"You mean, how do I feel as in my feelings, or how does it feel as in my body?" If Missy was asking about his feelings, which was far easier to share with her than describing the way his body felt when his muscles were too weak to work properly.

"Well, if it was me, I'd be really upset that nobody could figure out what I was trying to say," Missy replied. "So I'm guessing that's probably how you feel in your heart. But I want to know what your body feels like so I can help you. If I know what to look out for, then I'll know when to go get Aaron or mom or some other grown-up to help you. I'm not old enough to get you the right amount of medicine, but I'm a really fast runner and plus," Missy added, "if I have to yell really loud, I'm probably the loudest yeller on the whole block."

"I know you are," Josh chuckled. Missy was a careful child who made sure she wasn't too loud when she played, but sometimes, when she was very excited, her volume control seemed to be set to ten on the proverbial dial.

"But getting back to your question about how it feels," he said, addressing Missy's question. "I guess I start sounding like Jar Jar

Binks or Elmer Fudd, and my face feels like it's getting pulled down to the floor."

He paused a moment to collect his thoughts.

"And my tongue starts to feel fat and lazy, and it doesn't want to move much, so it's like having a really big tongue depressor in my mouth."

Missy made a face. She hated the taste and feel of tongue depressors, and she couldn't imagine an entire tongue feeling like one.

"My throat starts to ache, and even if I start talking at a normal volume, by the end of the sentence, there's no volume left at all. The best way to describe is like this: The longer I talk, the more it feels like I'm wearing a shirt with a collar that keeps on shrinking."

"It probably hurts a way lot, too, right?" Missy knew how it bugged her to wear turtleneck sweaters during the winter months, so wearing one where the neck kept getting smaller and smaller would definitely be a terrible feeling.

"It does, but the worst part is that my voice sounds weird," Josh shared. "It gets all up in my nose and pitchy."

"Pitchy, like the singers on those singing competition shows on television?" Missy asked, thinking of few times her mother had let her watch the finals where the winner was finally chosen.

"Yeah, pitchy like that," Josh laughed. Missy had a way of putting things together in her head that no one else would think of, and it always seemed to make sense in the end.

"So if you start talking like your face is falling off and your tongue is too big for your mouth and your throat hurts and your words disappear, that's stuff I should look out for, right?" Missy asked, stringing all the information into one long sentence.

"Pretty much," Josh confirmed.

Just then, Aaron reappeared with three glasses of ice cold lemonade with ice cubes clinking about, and lemon wedges floating on top.

"I think we should call it a day with the basketball," Aaron announced as he handed Josh a glass.

"Scared I might catch up and beat you?" Josh joked, as he winked at Missy.

"Yeah, scared he might catch up and beat you, Aaron?" Missy repeated with a grin, joining in the teasing.

"Tired is all," Aaron replied. "I think I've had enough exercise for the day. Besides, I've got work to do. That job I'm doing for Roy isn't going to get done all by itself, you know."

"No problem," Josh told his older brother. "We can pick up where we left off tomorrow or the day after …"

"Or even the day after that," Missy interrupted.

"Later 'gator," Aaron said as he stepped back inside.

"In a while, crocodile," Missy rejoined before dissolving into a fit of laughter.

CHAPTER 3

As she recovered from her laughing fit, Missy decided that this was as good a time as any to get lots of answers from Josh about Myasthenia Gravis. After all, the basketball game had come to a sudden ending, and there was a lot of afternoon left before mom called them in for dinner.

"You know that fat tongue thing you mentioned?" she began.

Josh's right eyebrow went up as he gave his sister a sideways glance. "Yeah, what about it?"

"Well, do you sometimes get a fat tongue when you're eating and that's why you always have so much ketchup on your plate?" she asked. "Or do you just love ketchup so much that you've got to have it on pretty much everything?"

Like most of his friends, Josh liked slathering ketchup onto nearly everything he ate. It didn't matter if it was French fries or eggs and sausage – with the eggs served sunny side up, of course – or ham, all alone or in a sandwich. He liked ketchup so much he even liked ketchup sandwiches!

"It's a bit of both," he admitted as much to himself as to Missy. "If you ask mom, she'll tell you that when I was little, she couldn't keep enough ketchup in the house."

"And that's why she buys the big restaurant size ketchup tub at the grocery store, right?" Missy interrupted. "The one that says it has a hundred and fourteen ounces in it that I can hardly pick up without dropping?"

"Probably," Josh agreed. He hadn't thought about it before, but it made sense that if a mom had a kid like him that ate as much ketchup as he did, she'd start buying it in bulk instead of picking up one or two of the delicate eight ounce bottles Grandma set out for dinner guests.

"Besides, if you're going to have M.G., you should make the most of it, don't you think, Missy?" he asked his sister in return.

Missy was confused. She wasn't sure how ketchup could make her brother's diagnosis better, but if he said it did, it must. Still, if she was going to get what he meant, she thought it would be a good idea to clear up the confusion sooner rather than later.

"I don't get what you mean," was all she said, hoping Josh would understand that meant he should add a few more details to the conversation.

"Well," Josh answered, "it's like this, Missy. Ketchup makes everything delicious, so that's not even up for discussion."

"Yeah, Grandpa says you eat so much ketchup, you should just drink it right out of the bottle!" Missy giggled. She slapped her right thigh hard with her hand the way she'd seen her Grandpa and Uncle Bob do when they said something funny.

"When I first got diagnosed when I was just a little kid, and way younger than you," Josh explained once Missy's laughter subsided, "the neurologist said that if I was having trouble swallowing, ketchup would make everything slide down my throat easier. And since I already loved ketchup, that wasn't a problem for me."

"Is that how come Grandpa says what he says about you and ketchup?" Missy wondered aloud.

"No, he says that because he's being funny," Josh chortled. "That's just the way grandpas are."

The cat that had crossed into Mrs. Whittington's garden earlier made an appearance as he traipsed back across their front lawn, and across the street before disappearing from view. Missy wondered if the cat was patrolling the neighborhood or just visiting friends and getting free tuna going house to house.

"Josh, if you liked mustard the way you love ketchup, do you think the doctor would've told you to eat lots of mustard with everything instead?" Missy asked.

Josh considered the question carefully before answering. It seemed likely that what was true of ketchup was true of mustard since they were about the same consistency. He just couldn't imagine anyone putting mustard on eggs and sausage, or French fries.

"I suppose," he finally replied, "if you thought mustard was way better than ketchup, which it isn't. It would probably work the same and help food kind of just slide down your throat and land in your stomach."

"Do you remember the limerick Grandpa made up for you that one time when we were at a picnic on holidays?" Missy tossed out.

He did, and, standing up, he struck a pose he thought transformed him into the image of an actor reciting lines on stage in a play by the immortal bard (as his English teacher called him), William Shakespeare. He sucked his stomach in and thrust his chest out. He imagined that at best, he looked like the actor who played Obi-Wan Kenobi in the original Star Wars movies.

"Joshua Barrett claimed he never met
A morsel of food that didn't get
Ten times better loaded up
With gobs of delicious ketchup
To help it slip handily down his gullet."

Josh had to purposely mispronounce *gullet* to make it rhyme with *met* and *get*, but that was part of the fun of the limerick. When their Grandpa recited it, it was even funnier as he added gestures and silly facial expressions.

Missy squealed with delight and clapped her hands. Her eyes danced, and Josh took this to mean his performance had been a top drawer effort. He'd heard the expression *top drawer* used in the 'Thin Man' movies Aaron teased him about watching, and thought it was about time the expression became popular again. If nothing else, it sounded classy, and for that reason alone, it deserved a second chance.

"You should make a video of that and put it on YouTube," Missy giggled uncontrollably. "Maybe you'll get lots of hits on it, and then it would go viral, and then maybe you could, I don't know ... tell people how come Grandpa made that up, and why you made a video of it."

Josh felt like hugging his little sister. She was always looking for ways to help people understand what she felt were very important matters. One of those important matters was Myasthenia Gravis.

She didn't think it was important just because her brother was diagnosed with it. She thought it was important because it was rare. Not too many people had it. She also knew that not too many people knew what Myasthenia Gravis was, or how to help someone with M.G. if they needed help.

Missy had been very vocal on more than one occasion when they were out in public and someone sneered or snickered at Josh when his muscles got unexpectedly weak.

"Yeah, maybe I should do something like that and talk about what it's like to have M.G.," Josh agreed.

"Maybe I could help you," Missy offered, excited that she might be asked to be the director or the script writer.

"Missy, if I make this video, *you're* going to be in it with me," Josh promised. He wasn't sure what he'd have her do, but whatever it was going to be, it would be safer than having her behind the camera shouting out Disney movie style directions at him.

"I could be your trusty sidekick," Missy hooted excitedly. "I could be like Harpo, and you could be like Groucho. We'll have them rolling in the aisles. Just like Grandpa says …"

"Yep, you and Grandpa are always saying stuff like that," Josh teased Missy as he winked at her.

"Because people remember fun stuff way better than sad stuff or bone dry facts," Missy continued, ignoring Josh's comment.

Josh sat back down on the front step beside Missy, and put his arm around her shoulders to give her a quick, non-committal hug. He wasn't much of one for displays of affection, but sometimes they were warranted. This was one of those times.

"Yeah, we wouldn't want this production to turn out to be like some of the boring movies they make us watch in school," Josh said.

"Yeah, no flat, boring movies for us," Missy decided as ideas began to gather in her head. "We're going to make a great big educational movie, and maybe even a whole series."

Putting her hands out in front of her she said, "Josh and Missy Barrett present ..." She moved her hands apart as if she was pushing drapes out of the way to reveal a movie marquis. " ... a Josh and Missy Barrett production, based on an idea by Josh and Missy Barrett about ..."

Josh shook his head as he laughed silently at his sister's plans. If he wasn't careful, Missy would launch a campaign to turn this one-minute video into a Hollywood blockbuster. On second thought, Josh considered how cool it would be to choose the actor that was going to pay the role of Josh Barrett. How cool would that be?

CHAPTER 4

"I just got a great idea!" Missy said impulsively, slapping the front step with her palms. "Let's go get some ice cream. It's a hot day. You just got done playing basketball. I cut a coupon out of the newspaper for a free ice cream cone at *I See Delights*, and we can use it as long as we buy one."

Missy wasn't one for sweets unless it was ice cream. It had been that way since she was a baby. If you offered her cookies or candy or cake, she was just as likely to politely refuse as to politely accept, but when it came to ice cream, especially if it was from *I See Delights*, it was a given that Missy would be standing in line for a serving.

"I don't know," Josh hesitated.

"I didn't mean *you* have to buy one so I can use the coupon," Missy clarified for her brother. "I meant that as long as somebody bought one, somebody else could get one for free. That means all I have to do is ask mom for some money to buy one so you can get the free one!"

Josh chuckled. Although Missy was taking after their mom with keeping a watchful eye out for what she called decent prices and good sales, her deals always wound up costing somebody money even when it wasn't meant to turn out that way.

"Tell you what," Josh suggested. "How about you run inside and get that coupon, and let mom know that we're going up the street for ice cream. That way she won't worry …"

"And ask for money so …" Missy interrupted, pleased that the coupon was coming in handy. After she clipped it from the newspaper the day before, she had slipped it into her coupon wallet their grandma had given her at Christmas.

"No, I've got cash on me," Josh cut back in, "so don't go bugging mom for money, okay?"

"But I wanted it to be a treat for you," Missy said, jutting her bottom lip out. "I don't want you to buy your own treat with your own money."

"It's still a treat," Josh insisted. "I'll buy you an ice cream cone and that's my treat to you, and then you can get me a free ice cream cone, and that's your treat to me. Deal?"

"Deal!" Missy agreed before jumping to her feet and running into the house to get the coupon, and inform their mom where they were going. Missy had learned very early on that her job, as a child, was to make sure her mom knew where she was at all times, and she took that job very seriously, even now when she wasn't a little kid anymore.

The door slammed shut behind Missy, leaving Josh to watch the occasional car drive by as he awaited his little sister's return.

Shooting hoops with Aaron had tired him out, and he was glad that the game had ended abruptly because Aaron had work to do. He hated when anything had to end abruptly because of his M.G.

It wasn't that people around him didn't understand why that happened sometimes. They *did* understand. It's just that it was unfair that it had to happen at all. There were times it meant that a family outing had to be rescheduled or that he had to stay back while his friends went off to have fun together.

He remembered one time in particular, when he was eight or nine years old, where his complaints about being saddled with something as horrible as Myasthenia Gravis seemed to fall on deaf ears.

He complained that he didn't think anyone should get to do things he couldn't do when it was all M.G.'s fault he couldn't do them. He grumbled that having M.G. sucked all the fun out of being a regular kid. He griped about how annoying it was that Missy could run around the house all day and never have to worry about her legs giving out on her, and Aaron never had to worry about looking like an expressionless goofball when he was tired.

Everyone in the world had it better than he did. Well, everyone except other kids like him that were cursed with Myasthenia Gravis.

His mother had listened to him air his grievances, all the while nodding her head. When he was done saying what was on his mind, she picked up the book she had been reading – the one she had set down to listen to him -- and began reading without saying a word.

"Hey!" Josh had yelled loudly, and she looked up at him calmly. She waited a moment or two, then went back to reading.

"Hey!" Josh had yelled again, louder than the first time, and his mother stopped reading her book to look at him. This time, she looked at him twice as long as she had the first time before she went back to what she was doing.

"Hey!" Josh hollered a third time. "What's wrong with you? I just poured my heart out, and you don't care."

This time, his mom put the book down on the table, and said, "Sometimes you just have to accept that life happens, and we don't necessarily like it. Yes, it's not fair that you have M.G. but M.G. doesn't have to run your life for you. Only *you* can decide how to run your life."

He was shocked. At first he thought his mother was being mean, but the more he listened to her, the more he realized that this was what she called a life lesson moment.

"Josh, you can either let Myasthenia Gravis beat you into the ground," she said with a gentle smile, "or you can decide right here and now to make every minute of your life count. Even when M.G. changes your plans, you can either let it make you miserable or you can find a way to make it work for you."

That had been a major turning point for Josh, and he resolved right then and there to make every minute of his life count, even those minutes when he was laid up in bed and couldn't go anywhere or do anything.

CHAPTER 5

Josh waited patiently for Missy to come back out with her coupon in hand. Josh remembered when Missy learned her lesson last summer about stuffing things into her pockets when a coupon to upgrade a regular ice cream cone to a waffle cone had gone missing somewhere between the front door and *I See Delights*. Mr. Carter who owned the store offered to give Missy a waffle cone when she couldn't find the coupon in her pocket, but Missy had politely refused. The deal was that the coupon had to be properly redeemed to get the waffle cone, and Missy didn't feel it was right for her to get special treatment when others who lost their coupons had to go without.

Josh's legs were sore from running up and down the driveway trying to best Aaron at basketball. It was times like these when Josh had to carefully assess how tired he really was. That was one of those things he had to consider because of Myasthenia Gravis: Should he rest before moving on to the next activity?

It wasn't just exercise that could knock the wind out of him. Sometimes it was something as simple as doing too much work on the computer, tiring his eyes out. And sometimes he could go on a long hike that only left him regular, everyday tired. The hardest part was figuring out what kind of tired he was, and if it was M.G. tired, he had to adjust his day to accommodate it.

His eyelids weren't drooping, and he didn't have fuzzy eyesight or double vision. That was a good sign. Usually if he started having trouble with his eyes, Josh considered those problems as a possible early warning alert that he was headed into the Myasthenia Gravis zone.

His imagination threw him a curveball and he imagined a parodied *Twilight Zone* intro.

'*There is a medical dimension beyond the one most people know,*' Josh thought with amusement. '*It is a dimension as confusing as math and as unpredictable as the weather. It is the middle ground between up and down, and between "I'm okay" and "What now?" This is the spot we call … the M.G. Zone.*'

"Hey watchya thinking?" Missy asked, the door slamming behind her and jolting Josh back to reality.

"Nothing," he replied. If it had been Aaron asking, Josh would have repeated the prologue, since they were both old enough to remember the *Twilight Zone*. But Missy had never seen the show, and sharing his thoughts with Missy would have led to a long, drawn-out explanation of both the narrative and the series. Sometimes discretion was the better part of valor, as their grandpa liked to say, and in this case, discretion meant keeping his thoughts to himself.

"So, are you okay with going now, or should we just kick back on the front steps some more?" Missy asked. She didn't want to rush her brother, but time was wasting, and the best time to eat ice cream was in the middle of the afternoon in Missy's opinion.

Getting up quickly, Josh nodded and flexed his muscles, showcasing his biceps.

Missy giggled. "You don't walk to the store with your arms, silly," she laughed. "Show me your leg muscles!"

Josh posed as if he was the coyote lying in wait for the road runner to come racing by, which made Missy giggle harder.

"That must make me the road runner," she howled. "Beep! Beep!" She leapt off the front steps and took off at breakneck speed across the front lawn, before tripping, and tumbling to the ground. Josh hurried over.

"Are you okay?" he asked.

Missy lay flat on her back and looked up at her brother before dissolving into laughter again. "You look so worried," she said as she rolled over on her side.

"You'd be worried, too, if you'd seen yourself fall," Josh assured his sister. "You were all apples over feathers."

"Sometimes that happens," Missy said, getting back up on her feet and dusting herself off. "And I didn't even get hurt so for sure, apples over feathers."

"Maybe we should just take our time getting to the store," Josh suggested. He paused a moment before adding, "And make sure that you didn't lose the coupon when you crash landed."

Missy realized that the coupon had flown out of her hand, but a quick scan of the lawn revealed where it landed. Picking it up, she reminded herself that going anywhere too fast wasn't the best way to get to where she was going. Her mom sometimes said that Missy spent so much time with her head in the clouds that she was surprised her daughter didn't trip over chalk marks on the sidewalk. Missy was pretty sure her mom was only kidding about that. Chalk marks weren't dangerous.

"Can we have the ice cream at the store instead of walking back with it?" Missy asked. She didn't really care one way or another if they walked back with it, but she wanted Josh to set the pace since he'd gone all out playing basketball. She didn't want him to feel he had to hurry back if he really wanted to split the trip to *I See Delights* into two parts.

Besides, it would provide a perfect opportunity to have a nice long talk with Mr. Carter, the shop owner, if he wasn't too busy. Missy liked talking with Mr. Carter. He and his wife had opened *I See Delights* a few months after he retired from his job as a weatherman at the local television station. It seemed that no matter how many times a person went to his shop, he always had great stories to tell about the summer of this year, and the winter of that year.

Sometimes, if Mrs. Carter was at the shop as well, she would tell stories about what it was like being a speech writer. Some of the stories made the adults laugh a lot, even when Missy didn't understand the humor.

CHAPTER 6

"Hi, Mr. C," Missy's voice rang out as they were met by a blast of cooled air at *I See Delights*.   Mr. Carter peered over his reading glasses and waved at Missy and Josh.

Missy ran up to the counter and took stock of the different flavors of ice cream that could be seen through the display case glass. She liked how the flavors were arranged by name and in alphabetical order instead of by color.   It made for a rainbow effect that incorporated the cheeriness of the shop.

"Hi, Mr. Carter," Josh greeted the shop owner.   "I'll be treating Missy to an ice cream cone today …"

"And I'll be treating Josh to one thanks to this *I See Delights* coupon I cut out of the newspaper," Missy interrupted as she placed the crumpled coupon on the counter, edging it towards Mr. Carter with her index finger.

The shop owner picked up the coupon and slipped it into an envelope beside the till.

"I just opened a fresh tub of Oreo cookie ice cream this afternoon, Missy," he announced, remembering that this was one of Missy's favorite flavors. "And the chocolate chocolate chip is a big seller this week, in case you're interested."

Missy mulled over her options. "Josh should order his first seeing he probably already knows what kind he wants," Missy proclaimed as she tried to figure out which flavor would win out over all the others in the display case.

Mr. Carter turned to Josh. "All right, then. What'll it be?"

"You know me," Josh replied. "If I was a car, they'd call me old reliable."

Mr. Carter grabbed a cone, and, scoop in hand, dipped it into the tub labeled *Maple Walnut*. He patted the ice cream into the cone, to make sure it would stay put, and holding it out to Josh, he said, "I could roll that in some walnuts if you'd like some extra crunch."

"No, thanks, Mr. Carter. It's okay the way it is."

"And super delicious, too!" Missy inserted into the conversation.

Looking over at Missy, Mr. Carter asked her if she knew what she wanted yet, and she shook her head.

"Let me pay for everything now," Josh joked as if he was picking up the tab on a large order. "By the time we're done, maybe she'll know what she wants."

"Don't bet on it," Missy warned her brother. "There's a lot of great stuff in here, and sometimes it's just way too hard for me to make up my mind the way you can. And plus, sometimes if the ice cream melts on me and it gets on my clothes, if it doesn't go with the color I've got on, it looks, you know, not very nice."

Josh found it funny that Missy would worry about coordinating the color of melting ice cream to her clothes. After all, it wasn't as if she was modeling this season's hot fashion picks.

"Have you narrowed down your choices?" Mr. Carter asked. If the choice became overwhelming, he had two suggestions at the ready: One was a reliable stand-by that sounded fancy like French vanilla or Swiss chocolate, and the other was a reliable stand-by with a twist like Mint Chocolate Chip or Rocky Road. With choices like that, even the fussiest of customers was certain to hit upon a flavor worth their money.

"Not exactly," Missy said.

"Well, seems to me that you're wearing a nice light colored shirt, so might I recommend a nice French vanilla or perhaps a more tropical choice such as banana?" Mr. Carter proposed.

Missy crinkled her nose up at the banana suggestion. She couldn't imagine why anyone would even think that was something she would enjoy even though she loved banana bread and bananas all by themselves.

"Perhaps the French vanilla with some chocolate sprinkles on top?" he continued as he gently nudged her towards going along with his idea.

"That sounds really good," Josh said, bolstering Mr. Carter's efforts to edge her in this direction. "It sounds so good I think that's what I'm going to have next time we come here."

"Then I think that's what I'm going to go with," Missy finally decided. "French vanilla with chocolate sprinkles. But not too many because if there's too many, it's not going to taste like ice cream. It's going to taste like crunchy dessert."

"French vanilla it is, then, with a smattering of sprinkles," Mr. Carter announced jovially, reaching for another cone.

As Josh and Missy waited patiently, Missy leaned in to Josh and whispered, "I just want you to know that if I drop some on my clothes, it's not because I'm making fun of you."

"How would that be making fun of me?" Josh asked, perplexed by Missy's quiet admission. Sometimes Missy's reasoning was easy to follow, and sometimes it wasn't. This was one of those times when it wasn't.

"Well, you know," Missy said as if the secret was known to them but no one else in the shop. "Like with the marbles."

'Aha!' Josh thought. 'This has to do with the food problems again.'

There had been times (although they didn't happen often) when he had trouble eating without a mess, either because he was having trouble opening his mouth or when chewing proved tricky. Generally he knew better not to eat when he was having trouble, but every once in a while, when he wasn't paying attention (like when he was at an all-day family picnic) and he got overtired, stuff happened.

He had taken to lugging around a backpack with a few essentials: a fresh t-shirt, a neck wrap that could be soaked in cold water for five minutes and wrapped around his neck or forehead to help him cool down, extra medication just in case, and other assorted items.

He couldn't lay claim to the idea of carrying around the extras. Their mom had come up with the idea when his brother Aaron was little, and as each child was born, a new backpack was put together and was placed in the front closet in case one of them had to be rushed off to the hospital.

"There you go, Missy," Mr. Carter said as he handed the treat across the display and into Missy's waiting hands.

"You should take a picture of this and put it up on Facebook," Missy proclaimed. "This is a masterpiece!"

"A masterpiece, you say?" Mr. Carter chortled. "Missy, if I had a camera, I might do just that."

"You can do just that with a cellphone because they all take pictures now," Missy insisted. She had a natural flair for marketing just like her mother. "And you don't have to put me in the picture either. Just take a close-up of how beautiful this is and write something neat to make people want to come down here right away and get one all their own."

"I'm afraid I wouldn't know what to say," Mr. Carter admitted, although he had an idea what he might write as a blurb.

"You used to be our weatherman on TV," Missy blurted out, "so maybe you could write something like: There's a cold French Vanilla front sweeping through the region with occasional chocolate sprinkles. Don't wait for news at eleven. Drop by *I See Delights* for on-the-spot updates. Paying customers always welcome."

Mr. Carter and Josh had to admit that Missy's blurb had the undeniable Barrett family marketing flair, and a knowing look passed between them. What Mr. Carter found especially humorous was the comment about paying customers.

"Well, Missy, how about we sit down inside instead of outside this time, and take our time enjoying our cones," Josh proposed. He felt some tingling in his legs, and resting would most likely take care of that. He savored the first few licks of the Maple Walnut in silence before Missy spoke again.

"I think I should ask Mr. Carter for a glass of cold water just in case."

"Why? Are you thirsty?"

"No," Missy replied. "I'm just thinking that if a walnut or a chocolate sprinkle goes down the wrong way, one of us is going to be coughing up a storm." She stopped and looked at her brother. "It's a just-in-case thing is all. I don't like getting stuff stuck in my throat."

"Yeah, that can be pretty annoying," Josh agreed. "But I don't think that's going to happen, mostly because I passed on the extra walnuts, but if you feel safer having a glass of water on the table, go ask."

"You never know when there might be a walnut piece that's inside the ice cream where you can't see it," Missy warned her brother, remembering the many times someone at the dinner table had picked through one of their mom's famous casseroles and found green peas mixed in with the other ingredients. The question was always the same: How did this get on my plate? And the answer was always the same: It must've been in the casserole dish when I made supper.

"You're right," Josh agreed. "You never know. So yeah, it might be a good idea, just to be on the safe side, to have a glass of water on the table."

He didn't really see the need for it, but he knew if he didn't go along with the idea, Missy would ask him about it every few minutes.

That was another thing about his M.G. Once he'd put aside some time to seriously think about his diagnosis, one of the things he realized was that sometimes people worried about him more than they should. Sometimes, they didn't worry enough. But that was okay. Unless someone actually had M.G. themselves, it was pretty hard for them to know when he needed them to help and when it was okay to just let him do things on his own.

It seemed to Josh that grandmas had the worst time of anyone figuring out when not to worry, and that was okay, too, because that's just how grandmas were.   Having a health issue wasn't what decided for grandmas if they were going to worry or just let things go. Grandmas, like moms, tended to worry maybe a little more than they should.

Overall, Josh had come to learn that sometimes it was easier to go with one of their mom's favorite sayings: Better to have it and not need it, than need it and not have it.

Handing her cone over to Josh to hold for her, Missy scampered back up to the display case.   A minute later, she returned with a plastic cup with ice cubes and water.

"Mr. Carter says if we need more water, he's got lots of wintery cold water in his fridge," Missy reported.   "I told him about the walnuts and sprinkles stuck in the throat problem that could maybe happen to you or to me, and he said that if that happened, he would bring more water to the table without me even asking for it."

CHAPTER 7

Josh and Missy sat silently, side by side, enjoying their ice cream as people filed in and placed their orders. It was turning out to be one of the hottest days yet, and business in the shop was brisk.

"Do you remember that time when you got to go in a helicopter to the hospital in the big city?" Missy asked as she watched the parade of customers wander by with single and double scoop ice cream cones, sundaes, and milkshakes in their hands and smiles on their faces.

Josh had been airlifted from the local hospital to the larger hospital in the big city three times that he could remember, and each time had been what the doctors called a Myasthenic crisis. As far as Josh was concerned, the reason doctors gave for being sent to the big city always sounded worse to him than it was.

That didn't mean that the situation wasn't serious, because it *was* serious, otherwise his mom wouldn't have rushed him to the local hospital and wheeled him into the emergency room. But Josh also knew that the doctors had specialties, and sometimes what M.G. threw at them wasn't in their comfort zone. Whenever that happened, that meant that his brand of Myasthenia Gravis needed other specialists to step in and wrestle it back down, and that meant he had to be sent to where those doctors worked.

Each time he had been airlifted to the hospital in the big city, his mom had gone with him in the helicopter, and Aaron and Missy had stayed home in the care of family and friends. After a few days, the doctors in the big city would announce that everything was fine again, and he and his mom would return home, usually by train (since the family car was driven back home by Roy and parked in the driveway at home when that happened).

"Yeah, I remember," Josh answered.

"And remember we had this really humongous big party for you when you came back?" Missy asked further.

It was hard to forget Missy's celebrations as they were usually very colorful and vibrant and yet, mindful of how tiring they might be to others. They came complete with pink lemonade, cheese balls, and pretzels as party refreshments, and a handmade *Get Well Soon* card signed by as many people as Missy could talk into signing it.

"Missy, you're not planning another party, are you?" Josh teased his little sister. He didn't think she was, seeing as he couldn't imagine any reason, but with Missy, it was always a good idea to ask just in case. She had a way of finding all kinds of reasons to pull together a party. Josh bit into his cone.

"Not that I know of," she replied nonchalantly.

Josh grinned. Whenever Missy answered that way, he knew that she was on the lookout for a reason to throw a party. Just because she didn't have a reason yet didn't mean she wouldn't find one in short order.

"Josh, can I tell you something I never told anybody else?"

Missy looked her brother straight in the eyes. Josh could tell that whatever Missy was about to share, it was serious business to her.

"Sure you can," he assured her.

"Did you know that I was scared every time you went to away in the helicopter?" Missy asked, glancing down at the table. "I was superly really scared. I was scared so much that I cried a whole lot until you came back home."

Josh stopped and stared at his sister. It hadn't occurred to him that Missy or anyone else would be scared any of the times he had been airlifted. But thinking back on it, how could Missy not be afraid? After all, each time he was rushed to the local emergency room, chaos ruled, with everybody doing something, and nobody knowing what was coming next.

"I know you were," he lied, hoping to calm her fears, "but you know, they sent me to the hospital in the big city because they know all about helping kids like me. And besides, they have more resources like specialists."

"But specialists are just doctors with more initials after their names," Missy said. "They don't just have M.D. after their names. They have P's and F's and C's and R's and stuff like that."

"Missy, when a doctor has more initials after their name," Josh explained, "it's because they did way more training than just to be a doctor like Dr. Henderson is."

"I like Dr. Henderson," Missy interrupted. Dr. Henderson was their family doctor. No matter who you spoke with, there wasn't one person who had a bad thing to say about Dr. Henderson.

"Well, think of the specialists like copies of Dr. Henderson except that they know extra stuff about certain things, like M.G.," Josh told his sister.

He paused and thought about how to phrase what he was going to say next to settle his sister's worries.

"Okay, so think about it like this. Aaron and I do stuff around the house," he said with a smile. Missy nodded. "And we know a lot about doing basic stuff like how to stop a tap from leaking and how to fix small engines like our lawn mower, but when it comes to the really big stuff, mom calls in experts, like a plumber or a mechanic. So the doctors at the local hospital take care of me most of the time when my M.G. is acting up, but sometimes they have to send me to the experts at the big city hospital."

"I guess that makes sense," Missy admitted, although she was still a little scared.

"It makes total sense," Josh guaranteed. "Think of a crisis like a really important football game. Before you scrimmage, you gotta huddle up and decide to have a play everybody agrees on …"

"You mean when they all go in a circle and talk secret so the other team can't hear?" Missy asked.

"Yeah, that," Josh confirmed, suddenly remembering that his sister struggled with sports comparisons. "So if the doctors here are like a team, and I'm like a football, sometimes the quarterback hands the ball off to a carrier to run with the ball, and sometimes the quarterback throws downfield to the receiver and he runs to the end zone for a touchdown. Either way, the goal is to win the game. The question is, what's the best way to do that?"

Missy giggled at the analogy. She hadn't thought of Myasthenia Gravis as being a football game, or of her brother as being a football, but it made sense in a comical way.

CHAPTER 8

"Just so you know," Josh whispered, as if they were undercover spies, "I'm not exactly fearless when *you* go to the hospital, Missy. Sometimes I'm afraid."

"When do I ever go the hospital for something scary?" Missy asked, thinking her brother was just saying this to make her feel better. She hadn't even had her tonsils out although lots of her friends had theirs out by the time all of them started kindergarten together.

"How about that time when we went hiking with Aaron not that long ago?" Josh asked, raising his eyebrows slightly, and giving Missy a knowing look. "Remember that time?"

Missy looked at her brother sheepishly. She knew what time he meant. It was the first time her brothers had included her on one of their afternoon hikes, and to mark the occasion, she had brought along the digital camera she inherited from Josh and snapped dozens of pictures.

When the trio came upon an abandoned church that had burned down, they noticed that someone had planted a garden and reclaimed the land. There were gourds and pumpkins growing on the ground, and peas and string beans crawling up the short walls that still marked where the building had once stood.

"That was the time I banged my head really hard on that metal pipe that was sticking out the side of the church," Missy said, making a silly face in the hopes it would take the sting out of the memory.

"That's the time," Josh chuckled.

"And then Aaron said, '*Hey, sounds like there's another church nearby; I just heard it bong on the half-hour*' except it wasn't a church that bonged," Missy continued, laughing at the memory of the mishap. "It was my head that bonged on the pipe."

"Yeah, one o'clock and all is not well," Josh joked back. He took a bite of his ice cream cone.

"It hurt so bad," Missy admitted.

"I'm guessing it did," Josh agreed. "Anyway, when we got you home, I was scared that maybe you got hurt way worse than you were telling us, and that was mostly because you didn't even cry after you got hurt."

"Well, I couldn't cry."

"Why not?"

"Because if I cried then I was going to scare myself," Missy confessed, "and I didn't want to scare myself. It was bad enough already that I got hurt, and Aaron made us go home right away instead of finishing up the hiking trip."

"Missy, he *had* to do that," Josh told her. "He was the guy in charge, and he had to make the right decision. The right decision was to bring you back home right away."

"Yeah, but that decision scared me and probably scared you, too," Missy countered, "so that wasn't *me* scaring you."

She remembered that Aaron had held up his hand and asked her how many fingers she saw, and when she answered that she saw all of them, that's when Aaron started acting like their mom did.

"Actually, Missy, I was worried after you bonged your head on the pipe, and scared when mom said she was taking you to the hospital," Josh owned up.

"But why?" Missy asked. "By the time mom decided to take me to the hospital, we were already safe at home."

"Yeah, we were home, but mom isn't the kind of mom that likes to rush off to the doctor with any of us over something she can take care of herself," Josh pointed out to his sister.

A dollop of ice cream fell from Missy's ice cream cone and landed full splat on her shirt. She looked down at the mess and pursed her lips. She had hoped to make it through her treat without what she thought of as a wardrobe malfunction. Now she had a great big sticky stain to contend with.

Josh picked up a paper napkin, dipped it into the glass of water, and handed it to her. She dabbed at the stain, managing to clean up the ice cream but spreading the stain in the process.

"Don't sweat it," Josh said calmly. "Mom always knows how to get stuff like that out in the wash."

"Except for when she doesn't," Missy countered.

"When she can't get it out, she does one of those artsy things moms like to do," Josh reassured her. "If she can't get the stain out, next time you put that back on, you'll probably have some embroidery right there." He pointed to the stain and grinned. "You know mom."

Missy laughed. Josh was right, of course. Their mom had ways to fix mistakes that most people would consider unfixable. Most times, the fix-it solution needed duct tape or olive oil, but every once in a while, neither duct tape nor olive oil would do the trick, and that's when the embroidery thread came out.

"But anyway," Missy said, abruptly turning the conversation back towards the previous discussion, "how come you were scared? I wasn't scared when we got to the hospital. Well, not too much. Okay, maybe just a little."

"Mom figured you might have a concussion from whacking your head so hard," Josh explained as he took another bite. "Concussions aren't something to mess around with, you know."

"If it was really bad, the doctor would have probably put a cast on it like you see on television," Missy replied in the matter-of-fact tone she generally reserved for answering questions at school. "In six weeks, my head would be all better."

Josh chuckled at the image of Missy wandering about looking like some Hollywood movie soldier with her head wrapped in bandages, complete with inconsistent memory problems, and Bob Hope or Danny Kaye waiting in the wings to perform a song-and-dance routine to cheer everyone up.

"Yeah, well, six weeks or six days or even six minutes, I was scared for you," Josh told her.

"But how come?"

"Because that's how it is in families," he explained. "When someone you love has to go to the hospital, it's just natural to worry and to be afraid for them."

Missy was about to ask why again when Josh held his hand up as if he was a crossing guard.

"Because that's what people in families do: They care about each other," Josh finished.

"So it's okay for me to be scared when you have to go to the hospital in the big city?" Missy asked, hoping she understood her brother's comments.

"It's okay for you to be scared," he repeated. "Just don't let it stop you from being you, and cracking me up with your jokes and stuff."

"Sometimes those jokes aren't on purpose, you know," Missy admitted as she ate the last of her ice cream cone.

"I know, and that's what makes them really funny," Josh said, reaching over and ruffling his sister's hair.

"Hey, stop that, Josh!" she said in mock indignation. "Maybe I could get another concussion from you doing that. It could happen!"

CHAPTER 9

Josh got up from the table once they had both finished eating their ice cream, and picking up the used paper napkins, he smiled at his little sister. It wasn't all that long ago that she had an imaginary world filled with make-believe animal friends and two imaginary characters that needed to be brought to justice: The Sneaky Itch and Floaty Penguin. Back then, Missy always insisted that Josh act as her assistant in much the same way that Doctor Watson was an assistant to Sherlock Holmes.

Now Missy was growing up, and sometimes *she* was Josh's assistant.

"I don't think we should drink the water," Missy announced. Grabbing the plastic cup, she added, "I'll just give it back to Mr. Carter to throw out instead."

Careful not to spill the cup's contents, Missy made her way back to the counter where Mrs. Carter had joined her husband a few minutes earlier. Josh watched as she handed the cup to Mrs. Carter, and engaged her in conversation. When Missy turned around, she was beaming. Whatever had been discussed, Missy was pleased with the end result.

"I told Mrs. Carter that *I See Delights* is the best ice cream place in the whole entire world," Missy broadcast. "It's important to tell people things like that but only if it's the truth."

"And is it the truth?"

"Is what the truth?"

"That *I See Delights* is the best ice cream place in the whole entire world?" Josh asked.

"It *is* in *my* world," Missy replied.

As they made their way to the door, Josh shook his head. Bottom line, Missy was right again (as usual) with her definition of what the whole entire world entailed.

They wandered slowly down the street in the direction of home.

"You know what I always wanted to know?" Missy asked her brother.

"What?"

"That IVIg you have to get sometimes ..." Missy's voice trailed off. She wondered if it was rude to ask questions like that, but she had questions that needed answers, and Josh had those answers.

"Yeah? What do you want to know?"

"I hate needles," Missy said as a precursor to what was to come next. "Doesn't it hurt when they do that to you ... poke you with the IV needle and then give you that stuff in the clear bag?"

Josh didn't care for needles either, but he also knew that needles beat the pants off having a Myasthenic crisis, and needles were a far sight better than being airlifted to the hospital in the big city.

"Here's the thing," he began. "I don't like needles. I never have, and I never will. But I like how I feel when I'm done getting an IVIg. I feel stronger and healthier and …"

"Like a superhero!" Missy finished for him.

"Not exactly, but pretty close," Josh replied, chuckling quietly to himself.

"Can I ask you some other stuff about IVIg?" Missy ventured to ask.

"Sure," Josh answered. "If it's too personal, I'll just make a face and say, 'Whaaaaaat?' and then you'll tell me not to make a face like that because …"

"Your face could freeze like that," Missy jumped in, repeating the phrase their mother loved to use whenever they made faces about eating cooked turnips.

"Yeah, that," Josh confirmed, making a silly face that made Missy laugh even harder.

"So does it hurt when the liquid goes in your body? And is it icy cold?"

Both questions caught Josh by surprise. He'd never really thought about whether it hurt or if it was cold. He was diagnosed with Myasthenia Gravis when he was seven years old, and IVIg had become an important part of managing and treating his case.

"I'll answer your second question first," he finally said. "For most people, their body temperature is 98.6 degrees ... maybe a bit higher for some and a bit lower for others, but 98.6 is the average body temperature. Pretty much everybody knows that. Even if you don't know how come, that's what doctors and nurses and moms always tell you is a normal temperature. So do you know how hot 98.6 is?"

"Well, it's probably really hot because in the summer time, when the weatherman says temperatures are going to be in the high nineties, pretty much every single grown-up hates that," Missy answered.

Suddenly, Josh threw his arm in front of Missy as they came to the street corner. He looked up and down the street, let his arm back down, and the duo proceeded to cross the street.

"So anything in the high nineties is really hot," Josh confirmed. "And if you have a temperature over a hundred, mom says you're running a fever, right?"

Missy nodded.

"So if just a couple degrees up from your normal body temperature is considered a fever, what do you think happens if you put something a couple degrees cooler into your body?" Josh asked Missy.

Missy considered the question for a moment, then replied, "Maybe it would feel like ice cubes are running up and down the inside of your body?"

Josh smiled, and nodded. "That's what it feels like to me … like ice cubes are running up and down my veins."

"That must feel terrible," Missy said.

"Well, it's not exactly terrible," Josh admitted, "but it's also not exactly tons of fun either. It just is what it is."

"And what is it?"

"Annoying."

They walked a few steps in silence as Missy considered what she had just heard. She had trouble imagining what it might feel like to have something cold running through her body, and admired that her brother didn't complain about ice cubes when he went for an IVIg treatment.

"But what about the needle?" she finally asked. "How much does *that* hurt?"

"Missy, I'm not going to lie to you," Josh disclosed. "Needles aren't any fun ever. But you know what?"

Missy shook her head.

"Once the nurse has that IV needle in place, I hardly feel it," Josh fessed up. "It's there, I know it's there, but it's taped in place so it doesn't move, so it's like it's not there at all."

"But you can't use your hand, right? You're stuck there with not moving your hand. Kind of like this." Missy threw her hands out in front of her as she did her best Frankenstein monster imitation, kicking her legs out straight as they walked.

"It's not like I can't move at all, Missy," Josh said, laughing inwardly. "I can text my buddies from my cellphone and stuff like that."

"Can you play video games?"

"As long as I have a WiFi connection and my trusty device, yeah, I can play video games," Josh assured his little sister. "Know what else I can do if there's no WiFi connection?"

"What?"

"I can read a book."

"A real live old-fashioned book?" Missy teased her brother. Her eyes danced with amusement. "One with a front cover and a back cover and a bunch of pages with black words printed on them?"

"I know, I know," Josh teased Missy back. "It's strange, but sometimes going old-school is the way to go."

"Oh, the shame of it all," Missy continued joking. "To think that all your techno gadgets may have to wait for the WiFi connection that will never come ..."

"Leaving me stranded on the island of Imagination where adventures and mysteries are bound to take place," Josh inserted. "I might even happen upon the elusive Sneaky Itch and succeed in bringing him to justice after so many years of bad behavior."

Missy rolled her eyes at the mention of her fictitious nemesis from her early years. In all the years she had chased after the Sneaky Itch in her make-believe world, she never succeeded in catching up with him and setting him straight.

"Missy, it's okay to have a great imagination, you know," Josh said, sensing that Missy might be embarrassed at the mention of her childhood adventures. "That's what authors have that other people don't always have. Great imaginations. So do detectives. That's how come they can out-think the bad guys."

"I know," Missy said, reluctant to admit that she felt silly whenever her past was brought up in conversation.

"In any case," Josh said, hoping his words would console Missy, "you're asking some really good questions about M.G. and I don't mind answering them. The more you know about it, the better you're going to feel about it."

"I know," Missy perked up. "That's why I'm asking you all these questions. Well, that, and plus I just want to know what to do if you need me to do something when your M.G. is acting up."

"Missy, you make being a brother real easy," Josh said. "You know how you're always giving out four-heart awards on your Facebook page? I think someone should give you a five-heart award for being you."

"I'm just being me," Missy replied, puzzled over why Josh thought she deserved an award when being herself was all she knew how to be. And besides, she was beginning to feel that Josh was very brave. Braver than she could be.

She wanted to tell him that, but she thought it would probably embarrass him, and Missy knew how much Josh hated to be embarrassed, especially out in public. She wondered what she could do to let her brother know she thought he was very brave. Maybe she could make a card and give it to him out of the blue someday. It would say *"To Josh! The bravest brother I know! Love, your sister, Missy Barrett!!!"* or something like that. The words weren't quite right, but the idea was. She'd probably have to sit down in her art area at home to work on the wording to get it just right before she started on the artwork.

The more she thought about Josh's card, the more she realized that she didn't want Aaron to get the idea she didn't think he was brave because he was brave, too. It's just that Aaron was brave in a different way than Josh. Aaron had *for-real* jobs, not just chores at home like Josh had and she had.

"I know you're just being you, Missy, and that's why *you* deserve an award," Josh exclaimed, as he elbowed her shoulder playfully. "When someone takes the time to find out what needs to be done so they can do it when the time comes, that person deserves a five-heart award. But that's just me. I'm not an award-giving kind of brother, so probably you should be getting a six or seven heart award."

"Maybe even a ten heart award," Missy suggested.

"Or twelve," Josh teased his sister. "But let's not get carried away or we'll be hearting each other for hours!"

"I heart you a bazillion million."

And Josh smiled.

CHAPTER 10

As they got within a block of home, Missy blurted out, "Oh no!"

"Oh no what?" Josh asked.

"The lemonade!"

"What lemonade?" Josh wondered aloud, his brow furrowing. They hadn't had lemonade at *I See Delights*, just ice cream and a glass of water that nobody drank.

"The lemonade Aaron came out of the house with," Missy wailed, distraught at the sudden realization that neither she nor her brother had remembered to take the empty glasses back inside before going to the shop.

Josh's eyes grew large as he suddenly realized that Missy was right. Those two empty glasses were still sitting on the front steps (or should be unless their mom had come out, seen the two glasses sitting there, and took them back into the kitchen herself).

"We're going to be in so much trouble when we get back," Missy cried. "Probably we're never going to get permission to take another glass of lemonade out of the kitchen again until we're ancient … like probably twenty years old or something like that!"

"Missy, we made a mistake. Mom gets that people make mistakes," Josh tried to calm his sister. "Besides, if we're lucky, she's been busy all day and hasn't had time to go outside."

"But what if she did and she saw the two glasses just sitting there, doing nothing?" Missy insisted on knowing. "And what if something bad happened? What if the neighborhood cats knocked them over and now they're broken all over the front steps?"

"Missy …"

"And what if Aaron came out on the front steps in his bare feet like he likes to do," Missy continued with the scenario, "and he stepped on the glass and cut up his feet so bad that mom had to rush him off to the hospital. And when they got to the hospital, the doctors decided to send *him* to the hospital in the big city and …"

Josh stopped walking, and grabbing his sister by the shoulders, he said firmly, "Missy!"

"It could happen!" Missy persisted.

"You're letting your imagination run wild," Josh told her, using the expression his mom like to use at times like these. "The worst that's going to happen is that mom's going to remind us that we can't leave stuff outside. The best that's going to happen is that the glasses are still out on the porch, so we'll just take them in when we get back."

Missy hesitated a moment, then the corners of her mouth began to turn up again.

"I guess you're right," she agreed. "And I guess Grandpa's right when he says someday when I'm a grown-up, I'll probably write lots of books and all because of my wild imagination! Really good ones, too!"

The duo started walking again, but it wasn't long before Missy had another question to ask her brother.

"Josh, you know how everybody tells me that when I go *what if* that I shouldn't do that?"

Josh nodded his head. One of the many things Missy was good at was imagining the many possible outcomes of any situation.

"And you know how Grandpa always tells me that if my *what ifs* make me worry, that worrying is like paying interest on troubles that probably never are going to happen anyway?" Missy stated.

Josh nodded his head again.

"And you know how sometimes my *what ifs* make me worry too much and I get kind of sick in my stomach?" she added.

"Yeah," Josh answered, wondering where this conversation was going.

"Well, mom says that when I get sick in my stomach, that's called stress."

"That's for sure what it is," Josh verified for his little sister.

"Well, I was wondering ... do you think sometimes stress can make your M.G. get worse?"

It was a good question, and one he hadn't thought about. He didn't spend much time wondering about the effects of stress, but Dr. Henderson had said – just like the neurologist and the occupational therapist had said – that stress sometimes triggered problems with health conditions like his.

"Dr. Henderson says that stress isn't good for anybody," Josh finally replied.

"But is it especially bad for you because you have M.G.?" Missy persisted.

"Here's what I know," Josh admitted, trying to put Missy's mind at ease. "I know that mom says she doesn't like stress in the house. Adults are always telling other people not to stress them out. Teachers are always saying that sometimes teaching stresses them out. And whenever you have lots of responsibilities at work, people say you have a stressful job."

"But what's that got to do with M.G.?"

"What I'm getting at is that stress isn't good for anybody, so I'm guessing that it probably isn't any good for somebody with a health condition," Josh said.

"But is it especially bad for kids like you because of the M.G.?" Missy asked again, rewording her question slightly.

"Missy, stress is bad for everyone even if they don't have M.G.," Josh continued. "But for someone like me that's got M.G., it's probably a really good idea not to put yourself in situations where you're going to get stressed out."

"Maybe you should get mom to home school you because school gets kids stressed out," Missy announced.

Josh wasn't certain if she was serious or joking. There were times when Missy kept a straight face while she pulled a person's leg.

"Mom's not going to home school me, silly," Josh chuckled. "She knows that home schooling would stress me out way more than going to school."

"No, I think it would be way less," Missy countered. She wondered why it would be more stressful to be at home than at school where sometimes kids could be mean and say things to hurt other kids' feelings.

"It would be way more because mom totally knows when I'm slacking off and blaming it on other stuff it isn't," Josh said.

"Teachers are easier to fool when I don't feel like doing something in class."

"Josh!" Missy said, shocked by her brother's admission that sometimes he faked how well he was feeling.

"It's true," Josh confirmed for his sister. "Sometimes I do. I know I shouldn't and if mom ever found out, she'd probably ground me off the Internet for a month."

"Maybe she would ground you off the Internet for *two* months," Missy said, her imagination firing up again. "If I was the mom and I had a kid that did that, I would probably break his Internet and say, '*No more Internet for you until you are so old that you don't live at my house anymore*.' And then there would be no more Internet until he was at least twenty-five years old and *that's* really *old*!"

"You can't break the Internet," Josh told Missy in a calm voice.

"Oh yes you can," Missy informed her brother. "Maybe you didn't see it on the Internet but there was this story about this lady and they said she put a picture on the Internet, and the picture broke the Internet."

Josh knew what Missy was talking about, but he thought it was best to let her think that the Internet had really been broken, and that some Internet specialists had repaired it. It was easier than explaining the meme to her, and explaining how a meme could jam up Internet traffic.

"But that doesn't answer my question: Is stress especially bad for you because you have M.G.?" Missy insisted on knowing.

"Yeah, it is. And it's also bad on other kids that have other health conditions," Josh finally admitted.

"Then you need to make sure you don't get any stress in your life," Missy stated with great conviction.

"Missy, there's always going to be stress in life," Josh told her gently. "What you have to do is try to keep it in check."

"Okay, then you better keep your stress in check," Missy advised him. "And I'm going to start by making sure we never leave empty glasses on the front steps when we go to *I See Delights* ever again."

"Good idea," Josh chortled as they walked up the driveway towards the front steps.

CHAPTER 11

"Josh! Missy!" a man in a blue F-100 Ford pick-up called out as he pulled into their driveway.   Missy looked over and smiled.   It was their mom's friend, Roy, who had known their mom since before Aaron was born.

Stepping out of his truck, Roy asked, "Is your mom at home?"

"She was when we left to get ice cream at *I See Delights*," Missy said quickly, as she stepped up on the truck's back bumper to spy at what was in the truck bed.

"Now Missy," Roy began, "you shouldn't ..."

"Woah!   Check this out, Josh!" Missy hooted enthusiastically, taking stock of the assorted wood pieces in varying sizes and thicknesses that were piled into the back of Roy's truck.

"You better step back down from there," Roy cautioned Missy.   "I don't want you falling down and getting hurt.   What would your mom say?"

Missy jumped back down onto the pavement.

"Thanks," Roy said as he winked at her. "And now, you said your mom was here when the two of you took off to get some ice cream?"

"Yes," Missy informed him, "but we didn't just take off. We had permission. Anyway, mom was here when we left, but that doesn't mean she's still here because maybe she isn't, but probably she is because I don't think she had to go anywhere today."

Roy walked with Missy and Josh towards the house.

"Josh, you know with Aaron in college now, I'm out an assistant," Roy began. "If you're interested, I have a job opening at the shop."

Roy ran a plumbing and heating shop in town that he had inherited from his father. Everyone in town knew Roy, and he was the business most people called first when they had work to be done in their homes.

"You should take that job, Josh," Missy insisted. The way she figured it, if Josh got the job because Aaron was in college, in a few more years when Josh went to college, she would get the job next. It made sense that the job would naturally be passed down to the next kid in the family (that being Missy) the way some kids were given hand-me-downs to wear.

"I'd teach you how to do basic plumbing and minor things like that, and you'd be assisting me when it came to more dangerous things like wiring and all that jazz," Roy explained.

"And plus," Missy added, "You probably get to wear a tool belt. And you can be just like a plumbing and heating gunslinger except with tools," Missy said, as the excitement built in her voice and her eyes grew bright. "You probably need a hammer for sure and some nails but not all the same size because not every job needs the same kind of nail. And you probably need pliers because mom says if you can't fix it with a hammer, you can probably fix it with pliers. I think you're going to need at least two screwdrivers, too -- one that has a star on the end of it and the other that just has a straight line across it."

"Sounds like Missy's already accepted the job for you," Roy laughed, winking at Josh. Josh smiled broadly.

"She has a way of doing things like that for other people," Josh chuckled and winked back.

"And you know what else you need, to be Roy's helper?" Missy interrupted, her enthusiasm running on high. "You're going to need a notepad and pencil. I have extra notepads in my bedroom and lots of pencils, so

I can give you a couple for sure as long as you let me read what you write in them so I know what to do when I get to be Roy's helper."

Just then, the front door opened and their mom, Jenna, stepped out. She held her hand up to shield her eyes from the glare of the afternoon sun.

"Hey, Roy," she greeted him. "And welcome back, you two." She glanced down at the front steps and saw the two empty glasses sitting off to one side. She raised her right eyebrow and looked at her two youngest children.

"I know, I know," Josh stated in a reluctant tone as he reached over and picked up both glasses. "We forgot. We weren't thinking."

"We were in a hurry to go for ice cream because it was so hot outside and plus, Josh played this awesome game of one-on-one basketball with Aaron, and he got some points and plus, Aaron quit the game and probably it was because Josh was catching up to him in the points department," Missy interjected, hoping her explanation would result in just a stern look and nothing else.

Jenna's face lit up as she looked at her daughter. It was difficult to be upset with her children when they tried so hard to follow the house rules. Most of the time, they did an admirable job. But sometimes, like with the empty glasses left on the front steps, they slipped up.

"Josh, I'll take those," she said as Josh surrendered both glasses to his mom's hands.

"I'm sorry we forgot," he apologized.

"I know you are," Jenna replied, her tone softening. And Jenna really did believe that Josh was sorry, not because he said so, but because she remembered the many times when she was his age when she forgot to follow the house rules her own parents had set for her and her siblings.

"Anyway," Missy proclaimed loudly, "Roy just gave Josh the job that Aaron used to have – well, that he still has now, but won't have much longer -- so now Josh is Roy's new helper at his work." She clapped her hands happily. "And we should probably have a celebration with maybe pizza for supper and more lemonade! What do you think, mom? And Roy can stay for supper, too, because he's part of the celebration!"

"Sounds like my evening just got booked," Roy joked with Jenna. "But just to be clear on things, I haven't given Josh the job yet. I wanted to clear it with you first. That's one of two reasons for coming over."

"What's the other reason?" Missy asked, curious to find out what was in the wind.

"Missy!" Jenna admonished her daughter.

"Well, Missy, the other reason has to do with Aaron," Roy started to explain before Missy jumped in again.

"He's working on that job homework you gave him!" Missy announced proudly. "I know because he quit playing basketball with Josh to go do his work for you."

Jenna gave her daughter a gentle warning with her eyes to let Missy know she was overstepping again.

"Mom?"

"Yes, Missy?"

"Mom, don't say yes for Josh getting the job until I get him a really good per hour money deal. I'm going to try to get him minimum wage plus one more dollar," Missy advised her mom, hoping that Roy wasn't listening too closely.

"Plus a dollar an hour!" Roy exclaimed, amused by Missy's plan. "He should be paying *me* minimum wage plus one more dollar with all the things he's going to be learning." Roy waited to hear Missy's response.

"Yeah, but, when Josh comes home from learning all that stuff from you, then he can tell me what he did and how you told him to do it," Missy replied. "That way, when I get his job, you're not going to have to teach me the same stuff all over again."

Josh looked startled, unsure if he should let Missy continue, or if he should stop her before the job went to someone else.

"That way, you'll get a way better employee right away when you get me. That means you're going to save time and money by not teaching me, and plus," Missy negotiated seriously, "when Josh teaches me what to do, it'll be kind of like him studying what you showed him to do already."

"I'm not sure that's such a good idea," Josh intervened, as much to safeguard the job offer as to slow Missy down.

"It'll be just like in that movie with that guy that teaches the other guy to yell, '*Show me the money*!' and the first guy wins the football game, and the second guy gets him the money, and after that, everybody's happy," Missy steamrolled on.

"It sounds good on paper," Roy admitted.

"Okay!" Missy said, confident that an agreement had been reached. "Let's talk out the details in the house."

Roy burst out laughing. "Like I said, it sounds like my evening's spoken for."

"Sounds like," Jenna replied as she turned back towards the house and held the front door open. Roy walked up the stairs and just as he was about to enter the house, Missy piped up again.

"Roy, what's all that wood doing in the back of your truck?" Missy asked.

"Well, I was going to take it to the dump seeing as there's not much I can do with any of it," Roy explained. "It's left-overs from a project I've got going over at the shop."

Missy knew that Roy liked collecting old wooden chairs, and that he kept them on the second floor of the building where his shop was located. Plumbing and heating was his job, but woodworking was something he did in his spare time. Sometimes, he even showed Aaron a thing or two about carpentry if things were slow at the shop.

"Can you let me and Josh have all that wood instead of the dump people?" Missy asked.

"It depends," Roy said, wondering why Missy felt the need to save the wood from its final destination at the town dump.

"Josh is going to help me build a pirate ship in the backyard," Missy announced. Josh's eyebrows shot up, surprised that his talents had been volunteered for a project he hadn't heard Missy mention until just now.

"A pirate ship?" Roy repeated, surprised (and at the same time not surprised) by Missy's plans for his discarded wood.

"Yeah, a pirate ship," Missy insisted.

"Missy, you're miles away from the ocean," Roy pointed out. "Besides there aren't any ships to pillage and plunder."

"Just because you don't see an ocean and just because you don't see any other ships, doesn't mean that something amazing might not happen," Missy explained. "If you stop believing in *what ifs* you might as well stop believing that fantastic things can happen."

Roy and Jenna stared at Missy, and smiled. There was something unmistakable about Missy's way of looking at life – simple and straight forward, and at the same time moving.

"Tell you what," Roy suggested. "I'll get Aaron to help unload the wood out back so you and Josh can build your pirate ship, and whatever you don't use, I'll take to the dump on the weekend. Deal?"

"Deal!" Missy agreed, sealing it with a high five, and without asking Josh if he had plans other than building a pirate ship in the backyard with her.

CHAPTER 12

Jenna pulled the door closed behind her as she and Roy went inside the house to find Aaron. Missy and Josh sat back down on the front steps, and Josh shook his head.

"What?"

"I know you're trying to help me out, Missy, but sometimes you just have to let me do things for myself," Josh said with a smile.

"If Roy gives you that extra dollar I tried to get you, for sure I think you're going to be happy about it," Missy replied, nodding her head. "And plus, it'll give you teaching experience and maybe that'll get you *another* kind of excellent paying job when you're way older and I'm working with Roy."

"Could be," Josh answered.

They sat quietly for a few seconds until Missy coughed nervously.

"Josh?"

"Missy?"

"I have one more really important question to ask you about MG," she said plainly. She paused a moment, then added, "Is it okay to ask just one more question? It's really,

really important and then I'll stop asking questions for today. Maybe even for the whole rest of the week."

"Yeah, sure. One more question," Josh replied. It was difficult to say no to Missy sometimes, and this seemed to be one of those times.

"Do you ever get mad because you have M.G.?" she asked timidly, not wanting to upset her brother.

Josh stopped short. Missy's question was an important question, and one that most people were afraid to ask. Nobody wanted to upset Josh by venturing into *the forbidden zone*, which is how Josh viewed other people's fear of the question that never got asked but everybody wondered about.

"Missy, sometimes I get really mad about having M.G., but mostly it's because there's nobody in the world I can blame in on," Josh finally answered. "Sometimes I'm mad at me because my muscles won't do what I want them to do … or what I *need* them to do. Sometimes I'm really mad and I don't even know why I'm mad. I just know that I'm mad and it's got to do with M.G., so to answer your question, yeah, sometimes I get mad."

"I'm sorry you get mad," Missy said, as she scooched over closer to her brother.

"But you know, most of the time I'm *not* mad," Josh continued, "and wanna know why?"

"Why?" Missy asked.

"Because sometimes you just have to buck up and get it in your head that things just are the way they are, and that's all there is to it," Josh stated firmly with conviction.

"You sound just like both of our grandpas when you talk like that," Missy giggled.

"Well, both of them know a lot of things, Missy," Josh readily admitted. "But you know, when you asked me about getting mad because of M.G., I realized that it's not any different than when I get mad at other stuff that doesn't go the way I want."

"Like when the TV listings say that a Godzilla movie is going to be on after the late night news, and you stay up just to see it, and then the movie comes on and it's something like a romanticky movie with Ooh-La-La Louise and He-Man Howard? And by the way, those aren't real actor names," Missy informed Josh.

Chuckling at Missy's example, Josh replied, "Yeah, just like having movies swapped out the way you said."

"I get mad when mom says we're having Sloppy Joes for supper and she makes hamburgers instead," Missy informed her brother.

"Missy, Sloppy Joes and hamburgers are both pretty much the same thing," Josh countered. "They're both made with ground beef, and they both get put on hamburger buns."

"But Sloppy Joes are fun and sloppy," Missy argued. "Hamburgers aren't sloppy."

"I can see your reasoning," Josh admitted. There was no sense arguing the point with her. While it was true that Sloppy Joes and hamburgers were nearly identical in most respects, he couldn't argue with the fact that Sloppy Joes were fun and sloppy.

"You know what's better than getting mad?" Josh asked Missy.

"What?"

"Doing something about it."

"I know what we could do!" Missy said excitedly as she jumped to her feet. "We could make the pirate ship in the backyard and let kids play in it."

Josh pondered how playing in a ramshackle pirate ship could do something about Myasthenia Gravis.

"We could make people pay a dollar for a whole afternoon of pirate fun, and then donate the money to a place that does M.G. research or that helps other M.G. kids! We could call it the 'Pirates, Parrots, and Poop Deck Party' and we'd let people know we were raising money for M.G. and everybody would show up and pay a dollar even if they didn't play on our pirate ship!"

Missy's face lit up as she began to formulate a plan to get kids and grown-ups to support her fundraiser.

"I don't know about the bit about letting kids play on something the two of us are going to build," Josh said, "but you know, I like your idea about having a pirate party to raise money for M.G. stuff."

"Okay, well then, we don't have to build one great big pirate ship," Missy was willing to concede. "We could build like two or three or twenty little pirate ships and paint them and stuff like that and then we could get downtown businesses to put them in their shops."

"How would that help?" Josh asked, baffled by the sudden turn Missy's thoughts had taken without advance warning.

"Mom could make a poster asking people to donate money by putting a dollar in the pirate ship at the store, and the poster would tell them to come to our pirate party, too!" Missy declared in swashbuckling style.

"Actually that sounds like it might just work," Josh admitted, realizing that Missy's fundraising idea had merit.

"We can get all kinds of people to help get the word out about our party, and then lots of people could learn all about Myasthenia Gravis!" Missy declared.

"It would definitely get the word out there," Josh agreed, impressed with Missy's off-the-cuff plan to raise money and awareness.

"And we have to have a reason to ask people for money -- more than just because you have M.G. so you have to tell me what would be the most best thing ever that could happen if we had lots of money to donate to a place like a hospital or something like that," Missy insisted. "So you have to tell me what the money we're going to get is going to do!"

Josh gave it a moment's thought, then answered, "I want it to go to research, to find a cure for Myasthenia Gravis."

"That's a great idea!" Missy smiled brightly at her brother, then added, "Make it so, Number One," in her best imitation of Captain Jean-Luc Picard of the Starship Enterprise. Josh chuckled as Missy dissolved into a fit of giggles.

Josh got to his feet. "Let's run the idea past mom first, and find out if mom knows any good carpenters to help us make those pirate ships you're thinking about."

"We don't need to ask mom about finding good carpenters," Missy told her brother. "We already know two!"

"We do?" Josh asked as he tried to figure out who they both knew that qualified for the job.

"Roy and Aaron!" Missy said excitedly. "Well, maybe not Aaron but that's because Roy didn't teach him everything he knows yet. I bet if we ask them, they'll say yes because I can't figure a reason out for them to say no."

"Here's the thing," Josh told his sister as if he was about to share a secret. "I'm game for going with your idea if you do the asking."

"You want me to be the leader of this idea?"

"Yeah, that's what I meant," Josh said, nodding his head. "I'm okay with you being in charge of the asking. Whaddya think? Deal?"

"Deal!" Missy agreed, putting her stamp of approval on her brother's suggestion. "We better pick a date and start planning this party right away so it's the best party ever!"

"For sure, this is going to be the best party ever, Missy," Josh agreed. He watched Missy as she skipped about on the front lawn. Who knew that answering so many questions would turn into planning a pirate party!

About The Author

Elyse Bruce does a lot of cool things. She's a musician, a composer, a singer-songwriter, a visual artist, an illustrator, a playwright, and an author as well as a mom.

She writes music, songs, short stories, novels and plays, when she isn't painting and photographing the neat things around her. She teaches songwriting and marketing classes at the college and university level, and leads workshops and seminars on a number of subjects.

Along with writing "The Missy Barrett Adventures" book series and "The Missy Barrett Conversations" book series, Elyse also writes the "Idiomation" book series and many other books.

She likes to create and promote new and exciting projects that engage, involve, and benefit as many people as possible. Just like Missy.

In her spare time, Elyse bakes chocolate chip cookies which she then generously shares with friends and family. Sometimes she even serves French Vanilla ice cream with chocolate sprinkles on top with those chocolate chip cookies!

Other Missy Barrett Books

Missy Barrett Adventures
For Young Readers

Houston, We Have No Problems
Guess Where I Am, Mommy
The Secret Ingredient
Foiled Again
Free Range Hiking
Nailed It

Missy Barrett Chapter Books
For All Ages

Roar Like A Lion
Fantastic Things

Missy Barrett Conversations
For All Ages

Barracudas and Impalas
Indians Live In Tipis

Missy Barrett Year In Review
For All Ages

The Year I Turned 8
The Year I Turned 9

Journals & Diaries
For All Ages

A Year Of Good Weeks

Visit Missy Barrett's website at
www.missybarrett.com

Follow Missy Barrett's blog at
www.missybarrett.wordpress.com

Visit Missy Barrett on Facebook at
www.facebook.com/MissyBarrettFanPage

Send Missy Barrett mail
Missy Barrett
c/o Elyse Bruce
P.O. Box 6306
Sevierville, TN
37864

www.ingramcontent.com/pod-product-compliance
Lightning Source LLC
Chambersburg PA
CBHW062042280526

45788CB00003B/1077